HARRIET ROTH'S

GUIDE TO LOW-CHOLESTEROL DINING OUT

A SIGNET BOOK

SIGNET
Published by the Penguin Group
Penguin Books USA Inc., 375 Hudson Street,
New York, New York 10014, U.S.A.
Penguin Books Ltd, 27 Wrights Lane,
London W8 5TZ, England
Penguin Books Australia Ltd, Ringwood,
Victoria, Australia
Penguin Books Canada Ltd, 2801 John Street,
Markham, Ontario, Canada L3R 1B4
Penguin Books (N.Z.) Ltd, 182–190 Wairau Road,
Auckland 10, New Zealand

Penguin Books Ltd, Registered Offices:
Harmondsworth, Middlesex, England

First published by Signet, an imprint of New American Library,
a division of Penguin Books USA Inc.

First Printing, September, 1990
10 9 8 7 6 5 4 3 2 1

Printed in the United States of America

CONTENTS

INTRODUCTION

When I learned that my husband had a coronary problem, I realized that we would immediately have to change our style of eating, abandoning the high-saturated-fat, high-cholesterol dishes we were accustomed to. At first we believed that "home cooking" would be the only road that could lead to this healthy lifestyle, that we would have to forget "the good life." After a few months, however, we began to miss the pleasures of dining out with friends.

Initially we approached the restaurant route very cautiously, limiting our restaurant choices to tried-and-true favorites where they knew us and would happily meet our requests. After a bit we became more adventurous and found that, if properly approached, many restaurants were very accommodating in responding to our questions and food choices. They even suggested options. Not only were restaurants becoming interested in filling requests, but chefs and restaurateurs were becoming knowledgeable about what low-fat, low-cholesterol cooking really entailed. They began to meet diners' needs for more healthful foods.

These days all of us know that it's important to keep our cholesterol counts down, but not everyone knows how to go about it. Fortunately, you don't need to be a medical expert to understand what to do, and happily, you can have a lot of control by making sure you eat the right foods.

This booklet will help you keep on the low-cholesterol, low-saturated-fat path whether you are eating out in your hometown, traveling by air, train, or on the high seas, or just "on the road again."

—H.R.

UNDERSTANDING CHOLESTEROL

Cholesterol is a soft, waxlike substance that performs certain valuable functions in the body. Cholesterol in limited amounts is not bad; in fact, it is essential to life. Our bodies obtain cholesterol in two ways: from the liver, which manufactures it, and from the foods we eat. While genes may determine how much cholesterol the liver produces, we do have control over the kind of food we eat. For that reason it's important to remember that cholesterol can only be found in *food of animal origin* like cheeses and other whole-milk products, meats, especially organ meats, and egg yolks.

But it is not just high-cholesterol foods that must be monitored. Foods high in *saturated fat* must be limited too, *for saturated fat raises cholesterol levels in the body*. In fact, eating foods high in saturated fat may raise your cholesterol even more than eating foods high in cholesterol.

Saturated fat can be found in tropical oils (palm, coconut, and palm kernel oils, and cocoa butter) and hydrogenated fats as well as in animal products. But saturated fat is often a hidden enemy that can take you by surprise, for it lurks in lots of foods, from various nuts and oils to baked goods and other commercial products.

Bear in mind that it is not the occasional indulgence that raises your cholesterol, it's what you eat on a daily basis. While you may find it easy to keep watch at home, if you eat out frequently you may find it harder to control your consumption of fat and cholesterol. And that's what this book is all about.

WELCOME TO HEALTHFUL DINING!

Today, much of our social life centers on eating out. According to the National Restaurant Association, Americans eat out about four times a week. While it is more of a challenge to maintain a low-cholesterol, low-fat diet on restaurant meals, there is no reason to feel condemned to sitting at home, forgoing the pleasures of dining out. All you have to do is find restaurants that offer you food choices that are healthful and then know what those selections are and make them.

Part of the joy of eating out is trying new foods. In fact, if you've never tried different cuisines this is an opportunity to expand your horizons, and with this booklet you can learn to be adventurous without being foolhardy.

The first thing to determine is whether you are given to sabotaging yourself. Take the following quiz to find out.

1 Do you feel that a low-cholesterol diet just means avoiding eggs and red meat?
2 Do you refer to yourself as a meat-and-potatoes person?
3 Do you include animal protein at every meal and avoid whole grains, pastas, salads, soups, fresh vegetables, and fresh fruits?
4 Do you think of bread-and-butter as one word?
5 Do you have your salad dripping with salad dressing?
6 Do you make each meal "the exception" and choose fatty, fried, or heavily sauced foods?
7 Do you never miss the chance to have that rich dessert?
8 When you do eat fast foods, are they fat-laden ham-

burgers, hot dogs, fried chicken, fries, croissants, Danish pastry, malts, quiches, tacos, and cheesy pizzas?

9 Do you think fish should just be eaten occasionally and then only if it is fried?

10 Is eating out *always* a "special occasion" that gives you permission to gorge on fat-laden foods?

If you answer yes to some or all of these questions, it's time to make some changes when dining out. The guidelines that follow will help you.

GUIDELINES FOR EATING OUT

1 Try to plan ahead and choose a restaurant that has a menu that will give you choices—not challenges. If you are not familiar with the menu, call ahead to find out if suitable choices are available.

2 Take your time in looking over the menu to find the right selections, keeping fat and cholesterol in mind.

3 Don't be afraid to make special requests or inquire about how something is prepared. More and more restaurants are anxious to please their health-conscious customers; some even list suggestions or mark them (for example, with a heart, indicating an American Heart Association recommendation).

4 *Select foods that are grilled, broiled, boiled, poached, or steamed without any added fats.* Avoid foods that are fried or sautéed or that come with a cream or butter sauce (at least, ask to have the sauce served on the side).

5 Choose fish, turkey, or chicken without the skin, steamed or stir-fried vegetables, or pasta rather than red meat, veal, or casserole mixtures.

6 If ordering an appetizer, choose broth- or tomato-based soup, not creamed; request a salad with the dressing on the side—better yet, ask for vinegar or lemon wedges instead of dressing.

7 Keep meat to a minimum. If the portion of protein in the entrée is too large (bigger than a deck of cards), either share it with your companion or order a "people bag" and take it home. (Microwave ovens are great for reheating leftovers, as well as for cooking.)

8 Instead of a large entrée, order an appetizer portion—it's cheaper and better for you.

9 Whole-wheat, rye, pumpernickel, and sourdough are good bread choices. Pass up butter and margarine, or prebuttered rolls.

10 Choose plain baked, steamed, or boiled potatoes or rice—not fried or sauced.

11 Order vegetables without butter or sauce.

12 Request fruit or sliced tomatoes instead of french fries.

13 Instead of mayonnaise or butter on sandwiches, use mustard and/or tomato.

14 For dessert, choose fresh fruit, a fresh fruit sorbet, angelfood cake, or nonfat frozen yogurt rather than other cake, pie, or ice cream.

It all comes back to you. You can enjoy eating out without sabotaging your cholesterol count if you take your good habits with you to the restaurant.

HEALTHFUL TIPS FOR "AMERICAN" RESTAURANTS

I start out with regional American dishes and delicatessen foods because all across America these are the foods that most of us are eating at least once a week. We may be buying foreign cars, and certainly Americans are becoming more adventurous in eating out, but the food trend is still toward regional American. Moreover, wherever you live, you are sure to find restaurants offering typical American cuisine.

Unfortunately, many of the traditional down-home favorites should be forbidden foods, so here's some help in selecting the right dishes if you are watching your cholesterol count.

REGIONAL AMERICAN

ENJOY	*AVOID*
Breakfast:	
*Any fresh fruit or fresh-squeezed juice	Butter
*Stewed fruit	
Vegetable juice	
Hot cereal: oatmeal, cornmeal, or any whole-grain cereal.	Grits (because they usually come with butter and are high in sodium)
Cold cereal: shredded wheat, whole-grain nuggets or whole-grain flake cereal (no sugar added), all bran	Cold cereals that are sugar-coated
Nonfat milk (or at least low-fat)	Cream or whole milk
Nonfat yogurt (or at least low-fat)	Whole-milk yogurt

*Whole fruit is preferable because of its fiber content

ENJOY	*AVOID*
Egg whites or Egg Beaters omelette (no cheese or butter)	Whole eggs of any kind
French toast (prepared with egg whites and milk only and grilled without butter)	Regular fried egg-batter French toast
Whole-wheat, rye, pumpernickel, or sourdough toast	Corn bread, biscuits, muffins, or popovers
Whole-wheat or water bagel, bialy, or matzo	Doughnuts, sweet rolls, or coffee cake
English muffin	
Melba toast	
Jam	
Postum, tea	
Decaffeinated coffee (limit to one cup)	
Enjoy occasionally:	
Short stack pancakes (no butter)	
Waffle (no butter)	
Appetizers:	
Fruit cup	
Shrimp or crab cocktail with cocktail sauce	
Raw oysters or clams	
Soups:	
Clear broth	Any cream soup

ENJOY	*AVOID*
Manhattan clam chowder (tomato base)	New England clam chowder (milk base)
Vegetarian lentil, black bean, or split pea soup	Seafood bisque
Vegetable soup	
French onion soup (no cheese)	

Salads:

ENJOY	*AVOID*
Any mixed green or vegetable salad (with lemon or vinegar, or vinaigrette dressing on the side)	Mayonnaise-based salads, such as coleslaw, potato salad, tuna or chicken salad
Coleslaw with vinaigrette dressing	Macaroni or other pasta salads with mayonnaise
Fresh-fruit salad with nonfat yogurt	Cottage cheese
Tuna salad plate (with vinaigrette dressing on the side)	Waldorf salad with mayonnaise
Crab Louis (without the dressing)	Caesar salad (unless dressing contains no egg and limits amount of Parmesan cheese)
Turkey chef's salad (no cheese or ham)	

Entrées:

ENJOY	*AVOID*
Steamed clams or softshell crab (no butter)	Sautéed softshell crab
Broiled or steamed lobster (no butter)	Lobster Newburg or any other seafood Newburg

ENJOY	AVOID
Any broiled, poached, or grilled fish (no butter)	Fried shrimp, scallops, clams, or fish
Grilled scallops	Fried crab cakes or deviled crab
Seafood kebab	
Barbecued chicken (no skin)	Fish and chips
Roast turkey (no skin or gravy)	Fried chicken, liver, or pork chops
Broiled or roast chicken (no skin)	Fried croquettes
Venison	Chicken-fried steak
Leg of lamb (small portion, fat trimmed)	Lamb chops*
Turkey club sandwich (without bacon or ham)	Barbecued spareribs
	Bacon, lettuce, and tomato sandwich
Lean roast beef sandwich	Beef dip
Vegetarian or turkey chili	Chili with beef
Vegetable plate (no butter or cheese)	Macaroni and cheese
Baked or boiled potato	Fried or scalloped potatoes
Rice pilaf	Mashed, hash brown, or french-fried potatoes
Corn on the cob (no butter)	Pot roast

*If you do, order trimmed loin chop

ENJOY	*AVOID*
All steamed vegetables	Beef stew
	Steak*
	Prime rib
	Hot dogs
	Hamburgers
	Sausage, bacon, or ham
	Corned beef or roast beef hash
	Meat loaf
	Chicken or beef pot pie
	Welsh rarebit
	Any egg dishes
Breads:	
Whole-wheat, rye, or sourdough bread or rolls	Egg bread
	Cornbread, biscuits, or popovers
	Butter rolls
Desserts:	
Angelfood cake	Any pie or cake
Applesauce	Pudding or custard
Baked apple	Ice cream
Any fresh fruit	Brownies or cookies
Fruit ice or sorbet	Jell-O (empty calories)

*If you do eat steak occasionally, order top sirloin or filet mignon broiled with fat removed—no more than 4 oz. cooked. Order it cooked medium or well; the longer it cooks the less fat it has.

DELICATESSEN

When you think of eating in a deli, images of overly fatted, cholesterol-laden foods generally come to mind. Indeed, all too many foods that meet this description can be found in delicatessens. However, as in most eateries today, there are quite a few healthful choices to be made. For example, you can usually find a delicious homemade soup or slices of freshly roasted turkey breast. So if you find yourself in a delicatessen, enjoy the smells of the hot dogs and pastrami, but limit your selections according to the following suggestions.

ENJOY	*AVOID*
Breakfast:	
See Regional American breakfast, page 9.	
Sandwiches:	
Turkey breast	Matzo balls
Roast beef*	Blintzes
	Kishke
	Kreplach
	Knishes
Soups:†	
Barley	Noodle pudding

*If you occasionally lust for a beef sandwich, choose lean roast beef (not corned beef or brisket) and then eat only half. Better yet, if possible order a half sandwich. All meat portions—whether in sandwiches, salads, or entrées—are usually ridiculously large. Control what you eat by sharing or taking home the other half.

†Remove all visible fat

ENJOY	AVOID
Bean	All cheeses (including cottage cheese)
Beet borscht (hot or cold, no sour cream)	Hot dogs, knockwurst
Cabbage soup	Corned beef
Chicken broth with rice (no egg noodles or matzo balls)	Pastrami
Lentil	Pepper meat
Split pea	Tongue
Vegetable	Salami
	Bologna
	Ham
	Chopped liver
	Brisket
	Short ribs

Salads:

ENJOY	AVOID
Pickles or green tomatoes*	Coleslaw with mayonnaise
Any mixed green salad with lemon	Chicken salad with mayonnaise
Chopped vegetable salad with nonfat or low-fat plain yogurt	Tuna salad with mayonnaise
Fresh fruit salad	Macaroni salad with mayonnaise
Turkey chef's salad (no ham or cheese) (with vinaigrette on the side)	Potato salad with mayonnaise
Any raw vegetables	

*Avoid if you are watching your sodium intake.

ENJOY	*AVOID*
Miscellaneous:	
Canned tuna or salmon plate with lemon	Fried fish
Gefilte fish plate	Potato pancakes with sour cream
Baked salmon plate	Mashed or fried potatoes
Chicken in the pot (remove skin)	Herring in sour cream
Roast chicken (remove skin)	
Broiled fish	
Smoked salmon (lox)* (no cream cheese)	
Chopped herring* (no sour cream or mayonnaise)	
Baked or boiled potato	
Baked beans	
Kasha (cracked buckwheat)	
Rice	
Any steamed vegetables (no butter or cheese)	
Applesauce	
Baked apple	
Any fresh or stewed fruit	

SEAFOOD RESTAURANTS

The restaurant of choice for many people who are watching their cholesterol as well as their calories

*Avoid if you are watching your sodium intake.

is often a seafood restaurant. Recent studies have indicated that fish and shellfish are high in Omega-3 fatty acids that help reduce the risk of heart attacks and strokes. It is a good idea to eat fish two to three times a week.

However, seafood can be dangerously deceiving, because these dishes are often cooked by frying or are accompanied by butter or cream sauces. Ordered properly prepared and unadorned, seafood can be your best ally, leaving your cholesterol level (and your waistline) in good shape.

ENJOY	*AVOID*
Seafood gumbo	Seafood or lobster bisque
Manhattan clam chowder (tomato base)	New England clam chowder (milk base)
Shrimp or crab cocktail (occasionally) with cocktail sauce	
Mixed green salad (vinaigrette dressing on the side)	Coleslaw with mayonnaise
Broiled or steamed lobster or lobster tail with lemon	Lobster Newburg or any other seafood Newburg
Any broiled fish with lemon	Fried fish or fried seafood of any kind
Stone crab claws	Deviled crab
Steamed hard-shell crab	Sautéed soft-shell crab
Steamed Alaskan king crab claws	Crab cakes
Steamed clams or mussels (no butter sauce)	Clams Casino

ENJOY	*AVOID*
Grilled kebab of seafood, fish, and vegetables (no butter)	Fish and chips
Baked or grilled potato	Fried potatoes
Corn on the cob	Any butter or melted butter sauce
Rice	
Any steamed vegetables	

STEAK HOUSES

Those of us fighting "the great cholesterol battle" avoid steak houses altogether. However, there are times when it's the only game in town. The good news is that most of the food served here is prepared simply and to order, so that we can easily make special requests. And even in beef palaces times are changing; many now offer a choice of broiled fish or chicken.

Often a salad bar is available. If so, start with a generous green salad (dressing on the side). Enjoy the bread—no butter. Order a baked potato (pile on the chives and forget the sour cream or butter) and have heaps of steamed vegetables (no butter).

Just remember to limit the portion of your steak (to a piece *about the size of a deck of cards*). Order a lean cut (Select or Choice) with all the visible fat removed. Prime-grade beef is out: it has too much marbled fat that cannot be trimmed. Be sure no fat is added in broiling. Another tip: order steak cooked at least medium. The rarer the steak, the more fat remains.

The cholesterol in beefsteaks varies only slightly depending on the cut. The big difference is in the saturated fat and the calories. Here is a chart to guide your choices.

FAT AND CALORIE CONTENT OF BEEF
(3 ounces broiled; visible fat removed)

	Calories	*Fat (gm.)*	*% Calories from Fat*
Rib eye (Delmonico) steak	191	9.9	47
Rib steak (Select)	181	9.6	48
Rib steak (Choice)	191	9.9	52
Rib steak (Prime)	238	15.9	60
Porterhouse (Choice)	185	9.2	45
Filet mignon (Select)	167	7.1	38
Filet mignon (Choice)	176	8.2	42
Top sirloin (Select)	162	6.4	36
Top sirloin (Choice)	176	8.0	41
*Top round (Choice)	165	4.3	24
Flank steak (Choice)	208	11.8	51

*Because it is so lean, it is sometimes marinated in soy sauce or fruit juice to tenderize it.

 HEALTHFUL TIPS FOR ETHNIC CUISINES

As travel to other countries and emigration to the United States from other lands increase, so does the demand for "foreign" foods. In some ethnic restaurants selecting is easy, but in others it may be harder. To help you, I have provided lists of foods to enjoy and foods to avoid in a variety of these restaurants.

CHINESE

Although Chinese food enjoys a reputation for being light, health-conscious diners must still use caution. Opt for steamed foods over stir-fried, and stir-fried over fried. Avoid excess sodium by asking that foods be prepared without MSG, and limit soy sauce. Insist that the amount of oil in stir-fried dishes be limited. And as a general rule, avoid beef or pork dishes.

ENJOY

- Hot-and-sour soup (no pork)
- Sizzling rice soup (no meat)
- Won ton soup (no pork filling)
- Steamed fish, chicken, or scallops; shrimp or crab occasionally
- Steamed dumplings or dim sum with chicken, shrimp, or vegetable filling
- Chicken or vegetable chop suey
- Stir-fried chicken, seafood, or tofu mixed with vegetables
- Minced chicken or squab in lettuce leaves
- Vegetable or chicken lo mein

AVOID

- Egg drop soup
- Fried or stir-fried dumplings, fish or poultry, won tons, egg rolls, or noodles
- Spareribs
- Barbecued pork
- Egg foo yong
- Pork or shrimp lo mein
- Mu shu pork, chicken, or shrimp
- Fried rice
- Sweet-and-sour dishes (most have been deep fried)
- Lobster sauce (contains egg)
- Fried apples or bananas with sweet sauce
- Ice cream

ENJOY	*AVOID*
Mu shu vegetables Moo goo gai pan Any steamed fresh vegetables Stir-fried eggplant, bok choy, broccoli, asparagus, green beans, and/or mushrooms in light sauce Lots of steamed rice Oranges, kumquats, lichee nuts, or any fruit	Almond cookies and fortune cookies (read the fortune and forget the cookie!)

CUBAN, LATIN AMERICAN, AND CARIBBEAN

Typical dishes from Cuba, Latin America, and the Caribbean can pose a problem because they usually rely heavily on pork, beef, cheese, and fried foods, with few green salads and vegetables, although complex carbohydrates like beans, rice, and potatoes abound. Happily, the fat of choice in cooking usually is corn oil (but ask to make sure). Butter is used only on bread and can be avoided. Tropical fruits are generally available for dessert.

CUBAN

Black bean soup Chicken broth with vegetables	Any pork dishes Any beef dishes, including ropa vieja (shredded beef)

ENJOY	*AVOID*
Cuban salad (avocado, tomato, green pepper, and onion)	Fried liver
Black beans	Any croquettes
White rice	White bean soup with pork
Brown rice (white rice mixed with black beans)	Fried fish
Roast chicken with garlic and onions (remove skin)	Deep-fried breaded chicken steak
Chicken and seafood paella	Any omelettes
Grilled shrimp in garlic sauce	Fried yucca
Grilled plantains	Fried plantains
Orange or carrot juice	Cuban sandwich (roll with pork, beef, cheese and tomato—a cholesterol killer)
Fresh papaya or mango	Flan
	Natela (crème brûlée with fruit)
	Grated coconut with cheese
	Papaya or guava with cheese
	Mango and coconut milk shakes

LATIN AMERICAN

Vegetable, lentil, or pea soup	Any cream soup
Mixed vegetable salads with vinegar	Stewed tripe
Hearts of palm and tomato salad	Any organ meats
	Any beef or pork dishes
	Fried chicken or fish

ENJOY	AVOID
Steamed or boiled potatoes	Omelettes or soufflés
Any cooked fresh vegetables, including turnips, squash, sweet potato, yucca (casava root)	Fried potatoes
Rice	Sausage, ham, or chorizo
Rolls or bread (no butter)	Any fruit fritters
Cooked dried peas, beans, or lentils	Canned fruits in heavy syrup
Paella (no pork or chorizo)	Fruited milk shakes
Any steamed or baked fish	Ice cream
Grilled shrimp	Flan
Roast or stewed chicken	Coconut cake
Fresh fruit cup	Any cakes or pastries
Fresh fruit shake with water	

CARIBBEAN

ENJOY	AVOID
Conch (red) chowder	Any beef, pork, chicken liver, or goat dishes
Testones (grilled unripe plantain chips), with black bean dip	Bombas (shrimp and potato croquettes)
Grilled chicken and mango salad	Fried plantain chips
Tropical chicken (grilled chicken with pineapple and banana sauce)	Spiced fried pork chop
	Conch fritters
	Coconut shrimp

ENJOY	*AVOID*
Caribbean chicken salad with banana and pineapple (no coconut) in garlic vinaigrette	Banana fritters
Paella (no pork or sausage)	Key lime pie
Spicy grilled shrimp, crab, mussels	
Pineapple and onion relish (served with fish and chicken)	
Any grilled fish	
Rice	
Fresh fruit	

FRENCH

Coaxing low-cholesterol low-fat meals out of a traditional French chef can sometimes be a no-win situation. French restaurants offer the greatest challenge in ordering a low-fat, low-cholesterol meal, as butter and cream are still *de rigueur.* But attitudes are changing, so smile, persevere, and plan your order. Choose entrées that are steamed, poached, broiled, or baked and avoid sauce, or ask that it be served on the side.

Steamed artichoke with lemon	Escargot
Vegetable soup with pistou	Pâté, foie gras (goose liver), and caviar (an occasional serving of the latter is okay)
Consommé with julienne vegetables	

ENJOY	AVOID
Mixed green salad (no dressing; use lemon or vinegar)	French onion soup with cheese
Truffles	Cream soups, bisques
Salade Niçoise (no dressing; use lemon or vinegar)	All salad dressings
Steamed or grilled mussels	Sautéed fish or fish in cream sauce
Roast chicken (no skin)	Duck
Grilled, poached, or steamed fish, chicken, or scallops with sauce coulis (puréed vegetables) or sauce piquante (tomatoes, garlic, shallots, and vinegar)	Any organ meat such as liver, sweetbreads, or tripe
Stewed rabbit (no butter)	Rack of lamb
Fish *en papillote*	Quiche, cassoulet, fondue, or ragout
Quenelles (fish plus egg white), no cream sauce	Any cream or butter sauces, beurre blanc, or béarnaise, hollandaise, béchamel, Mornay, or velouté sauces
Any steamed or grilled vegetables	Anything served *en croûte* (in a puff pastry)
Ratatouille	Buttered or au gratin vegetables
Bouillabaisse (tomato-flavored fish stew/no *rouille*)	Brioche or croissant
Pot-au-feu (chicken in broth), with chicken only (no skin)	All pastries (Napoleons, fruit tarts), mousses, crème brûlée, crêpes Suzette, soufflés, beignets, and chocolate truffles
Bread (no butter)	Any cheese

ENJOY	*AVOID*
Poached fruit	
Fresh fruit or fruit sorbet	
Meringue shells with fruit	

GERMAN

In the average German restaurant, the attitudes toward food have shown little change. Far more attention is paid to dieting and losing weight than to a healthful diet low in fat and cholesterol. Butter and cheese still have center stage and heavy foods high in fat abound, while sausages and beers of all descriptions seem to be staples. In Germany, restaurant menus are required to publish the nutritive value of all foods listed as low-calorie items. Because of this requirement, many restaurants avoid serving foods that are low in fat or on the light side, so eating German-style food and controlling your cholesterol will test your skills.

Enjoy	Avoid
Muesli	Butter
Bouillon	Any egg dishes
Lentil soup	Any schnitzel
Venison	Sausage
Hasenpfeffer (rabbit) (no butter)	Liverwurst
Rice	Pork or veal
Cooked red cabbage	Meat loaf or meatballs
Any mixed vegetable salad (no mayonnaise)	Spaetzle (egg dumplings)
Potato salad (no bacon)	Schlag (whipped cream)
	Kuchen, kugelhopf
	Black Forest cake

ENJOY	*AVOID*
All fresh vegetables (no butter or sauce)	Any other cake (particularly cheese) or pastries
Any breads	Strudel
Fruit compote	Butter cookies
	Fritters

INDIAN

Here the abundance of vegetables, lentils, grains, and yogurt that are typical simplifies ordering low-fat, low-cholesterol meals. The use of spices adds variety and flavor to Indian food, but be sure to inquire as to whether coconut oil or coconut milk has been used in preparing the curries. Choose dishes that offer limited portions of chicken (without the skin) and fish.

Mulligatawny soup (chicken with lentils)	Curries made with coconut milk or cream
Dal (lentils)	Vegetable korma (cooked with cream and nuts)
Vegetable curries	Puri and paratha (fried breads)
Aloo chole (chickpeas with tomato and potato)	Beef or lamb dishes
Biryanis and pilafs (rice-based dishes)	Ghee (clarified butter)
Basmati rice with vegetables, saffron, or shrimp (no butter)	Samosa (fried vegetable turnover)
Tandoori chicken or fish	Shrimp malai (cooked with cream and coconut)
Chicken or fish vindaloo (cooked with hot spices)	Koulfi (ice cream with nuts)

ENJOY	AVOID
Fish masala (with yogurt sauce)	Gulab jamuns (fried milk balls)
Shrimp bhuna with onion, tomato, and other vegetables	
Masala dosa (ground lentils and rice grilled and filled with potato and onion or other vegetables	
Naan, pulka, and chapati (baked breads)	
Pappadams (lentil wafers)	
Tamariná or coriander sauce	
Raita (cucumber and yogurt)	
Mango, mint, or onion chutney	

ITALIAN

There is much good healthful eating to be enjoyed in Italian restaurants. For years, many people shied away from pasta as a calorie-laden food. However, we now realize that pasta itself (without added egg) is a great source of complex carbohydrates—it is the cream and cheese that are sometimes used which add not only calories but fat and cholesterol. Although the olive oil used in Italian restaurants is enjoying good press nutritionally speaking, remember that it still contains

120 calories per tablespoon, so ask to limit the amount used if possible. Remember, it's a fat, albeit a good one, so go easy.

ENJOY	*AVOID*
Antipasto (no meat, cheese, or anchovies)	Added Parmesan cheese on all foods
Zuppa de pesce (fish soup)	Stracciatella (soup with egg)
Minestrone	Prosciutto
Pasta e fagioli	Clams casino
Chicken broth with pasta	Mozzarella marinara
Steamed clams or mussels marinara	Mozzarella and tomato salad
Panzanella	Caesar salad
Marinated artichokes	All fettuccini (has egg yolks)
Roasted pepper salad	Pepperoni
Tomato and onion salad	Manicotti
Italian salad (without cheese or salami)	Lasagne (unless vegetarian with little cheese)
Tuna and bean salad	Cannelloni
Vegetarian pizza (no cheese)	White clam sauce (if it has cream added)
Bread and bread sticks (no butter)	Pesto sauce (limited amounts occasionally)
Focaccia	All dishes prepared Alfredo or Parmigiana
Bruschetta (garlic toast with olive oil)	Any deep-fried fish or seafood (including calamari)
Risotto (without butter)	
Pasta with tomato and basil	
Pasta with marinara sauce (no meat)	

ENJOY	*AVOID*
Chicken ravioli with marinara sauce	Spumoni
Pasta primavera	Censi (pie dough fried in lard and sugared)
Linguini with red clam sauce (or white clam sauce without added cream)	Gelati
Linguini with broccoli, garlic, and olive oil	Zabaglione
Polenta (without butter or cheese)	Cannoli and other pastries
Chicken cacciatore	
Cioppino	
Broiled fish with tomato-based sauce	
Chicken Marsala (no skin)	
Italian ice	
Fresh fruit	
Decaffeinated espresso or cappuccino	

JAPANESE

Among the peoples of the world, the Japanese have the longest lifespan; as of 1983 it was 79.8 years for women and 74.2 for men. This longevity is due primarily to the traditional Japanese diet, which is composed of small meals low in saturated fat and cholesterol (little meat, dairy products, or rich sauces). This may change with the proliferation of American fast-food restaurants in Japan and the resultant increase in the intake of calories, animal fat, and dairy products.

One word of caution: If you are hypersensitive, be aware that standard Japanese food may be too high in sodium because of the amounts of soy sauce, smoked fish, and seaweed that are used.

ENJOY

- Matsutake mushrooms with lemon (or in broth)
- Suimono (clear broth)
- Soudon (broth with noodles)
- Miso soup with fish or mushrooms
- Pickled vegetables
- Sushi
- Sashimi
- Sukiyaki
- Shabu-shabu
- Tataki (seared tuna)
- Chicken or fish teriyaki, broiled (yakimono), cooked in broth, or steamed with vegetables
- Yaki-soba (buckwheat noodles)
- Yakitori (grilled chicken)
- Tofu
- Steamed rice
- Menrui (noodles in soup)
- Sunomono (cucumber salad)
- Konyakku (yams)

AVOID

- Any beef or pork entrées
- No chicken liver, gizzard, or heart
- Tempura (fried meat, fish, shrimp, or vegetable)
- Donburi (rice dish with fried meat or fish and egg)
- Green tea ice cream or any other ice cream

ENJOY | *AVOID*

Momiji-droshi (grated carrot and ginger)

Kaki (persimmon) or any other fresh fruit

Green tea sherbet or any other sherbet

MEXICAN

Many people feel that Mexican food is out of bounds. However, if you can avoid those foods that are prepared with lard or palm or coconut oil, and stay away from sour cream and cheese, Mexican food offers some delicious choices. What's left, you ask? Read on.

Soft corn or wheat tortillas* with salsa or a bit of guacamole

Gazpacho

Seviche (marinated seafood)

Salad of mixed greens, tomato, and onion

Soft chicken taco with lettuce and tomato

Soft bean, vegetable, or fish burrito (with corn tortilla and vegetarian refried beans, no cheese)

Menudo (soup with tripe)

Appetizers such as fried corn chips, chimichangas, or mini tacos

Chili con queso

Chili con carne

Nachos with cheese and refried beans

Crisp fried tacos of any kind

Fried burritos of any kind

Tamales

Carnitas

Chorizo (Mexican sausage)

*Flour tortillas are generally made with lard and are not whole-grain.

ENJOY	*AVOID*
Chicken, seafood, or bean enchiladas with green sauce or hot sauce (no cheese, sour cream, or guacamole)	Huevos rancheros or à la Mexicana (unless prepared without egg yolks)
Shrimp or fish Veracruz (with tomato sauce)	Any enchiladas with cheese, sour cream, or guacamole
Arroz con pollo (chicken with rice—remove skin)	Chiles rellenos
Chicken or shrimp fajitas (grilled chicken or shrimp with onions and peppers in a corn tortilla)	Any dish with mole sauce
Mexican rice	Beef fajitas
Black or red beans	Refried beans with lard
Vegetarian refried beans (no lard) with salsa	Fried tostada
Chicken, vegetable, or shrimp tostada with soft corn tortilla	Ice cream
Fresh fruit or sorbet	Fried ice cream
	Flan or any other custard or pudding
	Sopaipillas (deep-fried dough with sugar)

MIDDLE EASTERN AND GREEK

In keeping with the Mediterranean dietary tradition, Middle Eastern and Greek restaurants usually use mono-unsaturated olive oil as the fat of choice. Obviously calories will count, but at least it's the "good" fat that you'll be eating. Healthful eating rules still apply, so avoid fried foods and any lamb dishes. Happily, with this cuisine you'll be able to enjoy a great variety of vegetarian and grain dishes.

ENJOY

- Lentil soup
- Greek salad with a very small bit of feta cheese
- Fatoush (salad of bread, tomato, cucumber, and green peppers)
- Minted cucumbers and yogurt
- Tabbouleh salad
- Chickpea salad
- Vegetable or chicken shish kebab
- Couscous, pilaf, bulgur
- Hummus (puréed chickpeas)
- Baba ghannouj (eggplant dip)
- Mujaddara (cracked wheat with lentils and onions)
- Sleek (kale, black-eyed peas, browned onions, and cracked wheat)
- Plaki (fish with tomato, onion, and garlic)
- Chicken lemonato
- Imam bayildi (baked eggplant with vegetables)
- Rice-stuffed grape leaves
- Pita bread
- Mint tea
- Fresh fruit

AVOID

- Fried cheese
- Grape leaves stuffed with beef or lamb
- Meat shish kebab
- Kibbeh (lamb and butter)
- Spanakopita (spinach pie)
- Tyropitas
- Deep-fried falafels
- Moussaka
- Shawarma (roasted lamb or beef)
- Gyro or souvlaki
- Baklava, barma, or anything else made from phyllo or butter
- Mamoo (fried short-dough pastries)

RUSSIAN

Unfortunately, Russian cuisine is largely devoid of vegetables and salads. By the time you read this not only will *glasnost* have affected the political climate in Russia but McDonalds will have opened fast-food restaurants there and in many European Eastern bloc countries, too, raising the already burgeoning fast-food consumption, to say nothing of the population's cholesterol levels. Here's some help in ordering in a Russian restaurant.

ENJOY	*AVOID*
Blinis	Blintzes
Limited caviar (fresh is better because of its low sodium content)	Beef Stroganoff
Borscht	Chicken Kiev
Any vegetable soup	Pirogen (potato and onion in pastry)
Yogurt	Shashlik (meat kebabs)
Roast chicken (no skin)	Any pork dishes
Grilled fish	Sour cream
Cabbage salad	Butter
Steamed or boiled potatoes	Ice cream
Chopped eggplant with onion	Babka (coffeecake)
Bread	

SCANDINAVIAN

Scandinavian food poses some problems because it relies heavily on whole-milk dairy products, particularly butter and cheese. Pickled and smoked vegetables and fish are ubiquitous—a problem for those who want to watch their sodium intake. Stick to plain foods and choose wisely at a smorgasbord.

ENJOY	*AVOID*
Muesli	Whole-milk dairy products
Nonfat milk or yogurt	Cheese
Lingonberry jam	Butter
Vegetable soup	Swedish pancakes
Pea soup (no ham)	Any egg dishes
Pytti panna (hash with chicken)	Salt pork
Pickled or smoked fish (limit—high in sodium)	Sausage or ham
Pickled vegetables (limit—high in sodium)	Veal, beef, pork
Poached or baked fish	Swedish meatballs
Venison	Roast goose
Roast chicken (no skin)	Any cream dishes
Gravlax (high in sodium)	Any fried fish
Marinated cucumbers	Any cakes or pastries
Any plain vegetables	Whipped cream
Limpa bread	Dishes prepared with isterflot, an animal fat, also used in candies
Baked apple or pear	
Fresh berries or any fresh fruit	
Jellied berry pudding (no cream)	

THAI

Generally, when we think of traditional Thai dishes, we envision foods fried in lard or tropical oils or prepared with coconut milk, coconut, or peanuts. In many Thai restaurants this is still true; however, there are many delicious dishes that you can safely order with occasional inquiries or special requests. Always ask what kind of oil is used in a dish; if it contains lard or tropical oil, pass it up.

Be aware that dishes adding fish sauces will be higher in sodium.

ENJOY	*AVOID*
Any salad (no peanut sauce dressing)	Any deep-fried or crispy dishes
Yum nuan salad (mixed vegetables)	Fish or chicken soup with coconut milk
Any *clear* soups	Crispy fried rice
Tofu soup	Any curry made with peanuts (also likely to use coconut milk)
Hot and spicy chicken soup	Any beef, pork, or duck dishes
Tom yum goong (spicy lemon grass soup)	Any dishes made with vital organs or entrails
Po tak (hot and sour seafood in lime juice)	Mee krob (deep-fried noodles)
Noodle dishes: ask that no egg be added to any noodle dish	Squid
Lardna (rice noodles with oyster sauce and chicken)	Added peanuts or peanut sauce
Grilled chicken or seafood (abalone, scallops, shrimp)	Coconut ice cream or pudding
Hang mung poo (spicy steamed mussels)	Thai custard

ENJOY	AVOID
Seafood with chili tomato sauce	
Prig king (chicken in red Thai curry paste)	
Pad broccoli	
Spicy green beans	
Assorted vegetable stir-fry	
Spicy tofu	
Tofu with bean sprouts and scallions	
Steamed won tons with shrimp or vegetable filling	
Ginger steamed fish	
Spicy steamed fish	
Spicy ground chicken breast	
Chicken in roasted curry sauce	
Garlic pepper chicken	
Steamed chicken balls with curry sauce	
Barbecued chicken (no skin)*	
Chicken saté*	
Steamed rice	
Ramutan (fruit)	
Lichee nuts	

Note: Since Thai spellings may vary from restaurant to restaurant, I give the English descriptions.

*Avoid if marinated in coconut milk.

TAKE-OUT FOODS

For those of you who are always racing against the clock, or perhaps just committed to eating take-out foods because of convenience, here are a few suggestions.

ENJOY	*AVOID*
Manhattan clam chowder (tomato base)	New England clam chowder (milk base)
Split pea, lentil, or vegetable soup	Any cream soups
Broiled or rotisseried chicken (remove skin)	Any creamed vegetables
Poached salmon or boiled lobster	Ribs
Cooked shrimp or crab	Fried chicken
Sliced turkey breast	Chicken or beef pot pie or stew
Chicken or turkey breast sandwich	Fried potatoes
Seafood salad without salad dressing	Quiche
Any vegetable or pasta salads lightly dressed with vinaigrette (no mayonnaise)	Cheese or pepperoni pizza
Stir-fried vegetables	Ham, beef, tuna, or chicken salad sandwiches (mayonnaise-based)
Pasta with marinara sauce or pasta primavera	Lasagne
Vegetarian lasagne (no cheese)	Pasta with meat sauce, meatballs, or sausage
Vegetarian pizza (no cheese)	Hamburgers
Corn on the cob	Meat loaf
Baked potato	Submarine or hero sandwich (cheese and meats)
	Potato, pasta, or coleslaw salads made with mayonnaise
	Buttered rolls

ENJOY	*AVOID*
Whole-grain or sourdough rolls	
Corn tortillas with salsa	
Pita bread	
Fresh fruit salad	
Nonfat frozen yogurt or fresh fruit sorbet	Garlic toast made with butter
Chinese food (see page 20)	Corn bread
Thai food (see page 36)	
Deli food (see page 14)	
Mexican food (see page 32)	
Italian food (see page 28)	

FAST FOODS

Like it or not, fast foods are part of our daily lives. Fast food may come from one of the thousands of fast-food restaurant chains or simply from those deadly local chow wagons that cruise your city. Americans spend over $60 billion a year on fast-food meals.

A typical fast-food meal consists of a hamburger, french fries, and a milk shake or soft drink. It may contain half of the RDA of calories and protein, *but* it also is loaded with saturated fat, cholesterol, sodium, and chemical additives to preserve, color, and otherwise ensure its uniformity, taste, and profitability. Unfortunately, most fast-food items meet this description, although some chains have now added fresh fruit and vegetable salad bars, packaged salads, and grilled chicken breast or fish in addition to beef and fried foods.

If you find yourself in a situation where fast food is your only option, turn to the salad bar or packaged salad but skip the dressings. If potatoes are available, choose a baked potato—not french fries or fried potato skins. Select roast beef over hamburger since it is lower in fat. If you do have a hamburger, choose a plain small one (not a triple-decker with cheese), and one that has been broiled, not fried. Pass up the mayonnaise or any secret sauces or dressings—substitute plain lettuce and tomato, or some of the vegetables or fruits from the salad bar. If chicken or fish is available, choose broiled or baked versions if possible; if not, peel off any breading before eating.

Forget all other fried foods as well as croissants, malts, and whole milk. If whole-wheat buns or nonfat milk are available, opt for them.

Obviously, you aren't going to die from an occasional cheeseburger and fries, but there is a way, when you have no alternative, to select intelligently in fast-food restaurants and get choices that are lower in saturated fat and cholesterol.

SOME WORDS OF ADVICE ABOUT FAST FOODS

1 The best breakfast is juice with cereal, pancakes (no butter), or toast or English muffin with jam.

2 Never order giant specials, and hold the cheese, sauces, and added bacon.

3 If you do order any fried fish or chicken, remove the skin and/or batter coating.

4 If possible, order a *plain* baked potato instead of fries. Arby's, Burger King, Carl's Jr., Dairy Queen, McDonald's, Popeye's, Roy Rogers', and Wendy's still use fat that is highly saturated—and raises cholesterol. *So hold the fries.*

5 Limit your shakes and soft drinks, because they are loaded with sugar, sodium, and calories.
6 Keep looking for fast-food restaurants that have salad bars (page 46) so that your ordering will be easier and more healthful.

DID YOU KNOW?

Taco Bell Salad has over 85 percent of the saturated fat that an average adult should eat in an entire day.
McDonald's McChicken Sandwich has more calories and fat than a Quarter Pounder.
Jack in the Box Ultimate Cheeseburger contains 15¾ teaspoons of fat.
Hardee's Big Country Breakfast has 280 mg. of cholesterol, over 1000 calories, and 1950 mg. (1 teaspoon) of sodium.
Dairy Queen chocolate milkshake has over 1000 calories.
Burger King Great Danish has as much saturated fat as an average adult should eat in an entire day!

AND NOW FOR THE GOOD NEWS . . .

All fast food isn't bad. For example, pizza, if you limit or cut the cheese, is fine. The crust is complex carbohydrate (a whole-wheat crust is best of all). The tomato sauce and vegetable toppings are also good. It's the cheese, sausage, pepperoni, olives, anchovies, and olive oil that are packed with fat, sodium, calories, and cholesterol. So if you do eat pizza, choose a thick crust and top it with loads of vegetable offerings and some sauce, while limiting or eliminating the cheese.

To help you decide what to eat, here are some "best bets" and their opposites!

FAST FOODS AT A GLANCE

BEST BETS* **(Leanest)**	**WORST BETS†** **(Fattest)**
Arby's	
Baked potato (plain)	Apple turnover
Roasted chicken breast	Breakfast crescent sandwich
Junior roast beef	Roast chicken club sandwich
Chicken breast sandwich	Bacon cheddar sandwich
	DeLuxe potatoes
	Super roast beef sandwich
	French fries
	Milk shake
Burger King	
Plain bagel	French toast sticks
Chicken tenders	Scrambled egg platter with or without meat
Chicken salad (no dressing)	Double beef Whopper with cheese
Small hamburger	Double beef Whopper
Whopper junior	Whaler fish sandwich with tartar sauce
	Specialty chicken sandwich

*Watch the cheese, bacon, sausage, mayonnaise, and salad dressings that are added to foods in fast-food restaurants—too much fat, too many calories.

†Be advised that most fast foods are too high in sodium; if you are hypertensive, pass them up.

BEST BETS (Leanest)	WORST BETS (Fattest)
	Croissan'wich with sausage or bacon Onion rings Great Danish Ultimate cheeseburger
Carl's	
Hot cakes (no margarine) Roast beef sandwich BBQ chicken sandwich Happy star hamburger Lite potato Plain baked potato	Bacon & cheese potato Super star hamburger Western bacon cheeseburger Filet of fish sandwich Onion rings Sour cream & chive potato Zucchini Sunrise sandwich with bacon Shakes
Dairy Queen	
	Triple hamburger Triple hamburger with cheese
Domino's Pizza	
12″ cheese pizza (1–5″ slice) Veggie pizza—no cheese	Any deluxe double cheese, pepperoni, or sausage pizza
Hardee's	
Chicken Stix Side salad Grilled chicken sandwich French fries (in vegetable oil, not beef tallow) Hamburger	Cinnamon 'n' raisin biscuit Bacon cheeseburger Big country breakfast Chicken Fiesta salad Sausage & egg biscuit Big roast beef sandwich

BEST BETS (Leanest)	WORST BETS (Fattest)
Roast beef sandwich	Fisherman's filet sandwich Mushroom and swiss hamburger
Jack in the Box	
Hamburger Chicken fajita pita Low-fat milk Club pita Grilled chicken filet sandwich Taco	Nachos Onion rings Mushroom burger Ultimate cheeseburger Bacon cheeseburger supreme Swiss & bacon burger Scrambled eggs breakfast Sausage crescent Cheeseburger supreme Mexican chicken salad Ham and Swiss burger Jumbo Jack Moby Jack Apple turnover
Kentucky Fried Chicken	
Mashed potatoes Baked beans Coleslaw Original recipe drumstick (no skin)	Buttermilk biscuit Kentucky nuggets Kentucky fried chicken Extra crispy breast, thigh, and wing Potato salad
McDonald's*	
Hot cakes (no butter) English muffin with jam Cereals	Big Mac Chicken McNuggets McDLT

*Look for posted nutritional information on all menu items.

BEST BETS (Leanest)	*WORST BETS* (Fattest)
Apple bran muffin Nonfat milk Small hamburger Chicken salad Oriental (no dressing) Chef's salad Shrimp salad Garden salad Lite vinaigrette dressing Sorbet	Biscuit with sausage & egg McChicken sandwich Filet of fish sandwich Quarter pounder with cheese Milk shake Apple pie Cinnamon raisin Danish Chocolate chip cookie Thousand Island, french, or bleu cheese dressing
Pizza Hut	
Salad bar 12″ cheese pizza (1–5″ slice) Veggie pizza—no cheese	Any deluxe double cheese, pepperoni, or sausage pizza
Roy Rogers'	
Roast beef sandwich, regular Baked potato, plain Hamburger Chef's salad Chicken sticks Garden salad	Egg and biscuit platter Bar burger RR Bar burger French fries Breakfast crescent sandwich with or without ham or bacon Biscuit filet sandwich Fried chicken Roast beef sandwich with cheese Strawberry shortcake
Taco Bell	
Chicken fajita Bean burrito with green sauce	Taco salad with shell Taco salad without shell Nachos

BEST BETS *(Leanest)*	WORST BETS *(Fattest)*
Taco	Beef tostada
Steak fajita	Beef burrito
Tostada	Pizzaz pizza
	Taco Bell grande
	Taco salad
	Seafood salad

Wendy's

Plain single hamburger	Bacon Swiss burger
Cottage cheese (½ cup)	Triple cheese burger
Plain baked potato	Taco salad
Side salad	Bacon and cheese potato
Chili	Sour cream and chive potato
Chicken breast filet sandwich	French fries
Small hamburger (Kid's Meal)	Frosty dairy dessert

NAVIGATING THE SALAD BAR

Salad bars can be a great source of vitamins, minerals, and fiber, but the dressings, cheese, bacon, eggs, and sunflower seeds, or the many mixtures with mayonnaise (macaroni, potato, egg, and tuna salads), can sabotage your well-intentioned goal of a low-calorie, low-fat, low-cholesterol meal. A ladle of blue cheese or Thousand Island dressing can add up to 400 calories to your meal, as well as fat and cholesterol.

Because in most cases you don't know the calorie content of the low-calorie salad dressing (if there is one), be on the safe side and use no more than one tablespoon. Better yet, use vinegar, lemon, or fresh salsa if available.

SOME SALAD BAR CALORIES

4 radishes	5 calories
6 cucumber slices	5 calories
6 green pepper slices	5 calories
½ cup mushrooms	10 calories
½ cup cauliflower	12 calories
½ cup bean sprouts	15 calories
¼ cup shredded red cabbage	17 calories
2 cups salad greens	20 calories
½ cup chopped tomato or 6 cherry tomatoes	20 calories
½ cup broccoli	20 calories
½ cup carrots	22 calories
½ cup beets	25 calories
2½ slices red onion	28 calories
1 tablespoon raisins	30 calories
½ cup artichoke hearts	32 calories
½ cup corn	40 calories
½ cup peas	60 calories
1 teaspoon sunflower seeds	60 calories
1 tablespoon croutons	60 calories
2 tablespoons bacon bits	66 calories
1 ounce cheese	112 calories (plus fat and cholesterol!)
½ cup kidney or garbanzo beans	135 calories
½ fried potato skin	154 calories
½ cup macaroni, pasta, or potato salad	175 calories

Avoid *all* salad dressings. If salsa is available, use that.

 BROWN-BAGGING IT

If you've decided to save your pennies, pounds, and time and pass up the fast-food establishments, try brown-bagging it. I'm not encouraging you to eat on the run, but for those days when you have to grab breakfast or lunch, try these suggestions.

Pack your meal the night before.

For breakfast, take fruit plus nonfat plain yogurt and a homemade oat-bran muffin or homemade granola (or commercial granola without coconut or oil added) or part-skim ricotta with a whole-wheat bagel.

For lunch, make a sandwich on whole-wheat bread or pita, using part-skim ricotta, a slice of light cheese, tuna or salmon spread made with yogurt, turkey or chicken breast, or a chopped vegetable salad for a filling. Or take a thermos of hot soup or cold nonfat milk, some whole-grain crackers, a salad mixture you've concocted from last night's dinner, and lots of fresh vegetables to snack on.

Note: If you have a microwave available at work, try baking a potato, steaming a package of raw vegetables, or heating some leftover pasta for a warm lunch.

For snacking, to kick the urge for candy or a high-fat snack, pack fruit—a banana, orange, apple, or pear, even a small box of raisins—and/or plain nonfat yogurt to fight that late-afternoon loss of energy and give you the boost you need.

ENJOY	*AVOID*
Fresh fruit	Whole-milk yogurt
Nonfat yogurt (plain or fruited)	Potato chips

ENJOY	*AVOID*
Homemade oat-bran or whole-grain muffin*	Corn chips
Granola (no coconut) or whole-grain cereal with nonfat milk	Store-bought muffins
Vegetable, pea, or bean soup	Doughnuts or Danish
Nonfat cottage cheese with vegetable or fruit salad	Cookies
Sandwiches on whole-wheat, rye, pumper-nickel, water bagel, pita, or corn tortillas	Fruit nectars
Filled with:	Candy bars
Part-skim ricotta mixed with chopped vegetables	Cream soups
Light cheese (1 ounce)	Carbonated soft drinks
Tuna or salmon spread (use yogurt)	Salami, bologna, ham, and other processed luncheon meats
Turkey or chicken breast	Egg salad
Turkey or chicken salad (no mayonnaise)	Egg bread
Chopped vegetables with yogurt	White breads
Eggplant or tofu spread	Buttered rolls
Some natural peanut butter with fresh fruit	
Crudités	

*Healthful quick mixes are now available

ENJOY	AVOID
Pasta salad (no mayonnaise)	
Salt-free vegetable juice, unsweetened fruit juice, or nonfat milk	
Rice crackers, Finn or natural Rye Crisp, whole-wheat bread sticks	

IF YOU ORDER DRINKS . . .

Dining out is often used as an excuse to overindulge in drinking as well as eating. By snacking on some complex carbohydrate foods like raw vegetables or crackers at home before you leave, you can slow down your appetite as well as the absorption of any alcoholic beverages you may drink. Alcoholic beverages, particularly many mixed drinks, are filled with empty calories, and excessive drinking puts on pounds.

Whatever you choose to drink, the following chart will help you see the approximate calories that reflect its alcohol and sugar content, as well as any other ingredients you might want to be aware of.

Beverage	*Portion*	*Calories*
Nonalcoholic:		
Mineral water with lime	Unlimited	0
Sugar-free tonic	Unlimited	0
Club soda	Unlimited	0
Diet soda	Unlimited	0
Tomato juice or Bloody Mary mix (high in sodium)	½ cup	25

Beverage	*Portion*	*Calories*
Orange, grapefruit, or pineapple juice	½ cup	60
Nonalcoholic beer	12 ounces	50
Alcoholic:		
Beer, light	12 ounces	95
Beer, regular	12 ounces	150
Wine spritzer (wine with club soda)	8 ounces	40
Champagne	4 ounces	84
Wine, white table	3½ ounces	80
Wine, red table	3½ ounces	76
Liquor, 86 proof (gin, rum, scotch, tequila, vodka, whiskey)	1½ ounces	105
Dry vermouth	3 ounces	105
Cocktails and Mixed Drinks		
*Brandy Alexander	1	260
Daiquiri	1	125
*Egg Nog (contains egg and cream)	4 ounces	250
Manhattan	1	165
Margarita	4 ounces	140
Martini	1	140
Old-Fashioned	4 ounces	180
*Piña colada (contains coconut and milk)	1	180
*Ramos gin fizz (contains cream)	8 ounces	260
Sangría	4 ounces	130
Tom Collins	10 ounces	180
Sherry (dry)	2 ounces	85
(sweet)	2 ounces	95

*These beverages contain alcohol and sugar, as well as the saturated fat from the added cream, egg, or coconut.

Beverage	*Portion*	*Calories*
Sweet dessert wine	3½ ounces	153
Port	1 ounce	50
Brandy	1 ounce	50
*Irish coffee (contains whipping cream)	6 ounces	165

*These beverages contain alcohol and sugar, as well as the saturated fat from the added cream, egg, or coconut.

The ever-present bowls of nuts, chips, or crackers served with drinks that you may have while waiting for your food—or your table—are loaded with calories and fat. If you find yourself in this situation, look for pretzels or unbuttered popcorn to satisfy the munchies.

THE LOW-CHOLESTEROL TRAVELER

For many people, the idea of vacation and travel means an automatic end to any diet plan. Maybe you agree. After all, you may say, how can I possibly control the food I get to eat on planes, trains, or ships, or even on the road? But I'll show you how you can keep to a low-cholesterol, low-fat lifestyle no matter where you go.

THE ONLY WAY TO FLY

When you book your flight, you can order a special meal through your travel agent or the airline (you must make your request at least forty-eight hours ahead of departure). Special low-cholesterol or vegetarian meals are available on all airlines. United Air

Lines offers an egg-substitute omelette for breakfast. American Air Lines has introduced "lighter, fresher, and more healthful cuisine" by serving sauces on the side, offering more chicken, vegetables, and pasta, and reducing the number of heavy beef dishes. However, since many of these meals are loaded with fat and sodium, I suggest you consider the fresh fruit, steamed vegetable platter, or seafood salad that most airlines offer. Ask for a roll, green salad, and beverage to round out the meal. If your flight also includes a breakfast, select fruit and cereal with low-fat milk if nonfat milk is not available.

Some of my clients have packed lunches for their flights. If the trip is relatively short, a sandwich, crudités, and fruit will fill the bill. Since on longer trips a packed lunch may get a bit gamy, it is probably better to choose from the airline's limited selection.

A bag of snacks—including whole-grain crackers, salt-free pretzels, popcorn, and dried and fresh fruit—is a good idea. I am happy to see that some airlines now offer boxes of raisins instead of those killer packets of high-fat, high-sodium, sugar-coated peanuts.

Because fluid retention can often be a problem when flying, drink lots of water or low-sodium mineral water and unsweetened fruit juices instead of alcoholic beverages, soft drinks, or high-sodium tomato juice.

CRUISING TOWARD HEALTH

In the past when you took a cruise, you had a fight on your hands. Cruises were often nothing more than food orgies. Today, you can consult your travel agent ahead of time to check out what your cruise line offers. Some ships provide low-cholesterol, low-calorie selections with healthful dishes on their regular menus, or they are pleased to honor special requests. Royal Cruise Lines has a program offered on all cruises called "New Beginnings" that has lectures on health and nutrition. In addition, the Royal Crown *Odyssey* has an American Heart Association–approved alternative menu called "Dine to Your Heart's Content." Admiral Cruise Lines has a separate menu page with Heart Association suggestions. Royal Viking has a spa menu geared mostly to calorie counters. Ideally, even if there is no special menu, most ships will try to accommodate your needs, since they have you longer than do the airlines. If the cruise you are taking does not offer these options, then choose simply prepared (broiled or steamed) foods without added fat, or refer to the various ethnic lists for guidance (pages 20–37).

Here's another tip: Change your focus and don't concentrate on the food. Instead, shift your attention to the activities, the people, the ports of call. Mealtimes can be pleasant social occasions, but after all, it's the change of scene and pace that you're paying for.

TRAIN TRAVEL IS BOOMING!

Americans' love affair with train travel is having a resurgence. The comfort, the wide aisles offering room to stretch and walk, and the constantly changing scenery have resulted in the greatest number of Amtrak passengers ever.

On short train trips pack a picnic lunch or snacks. On longer runs you will find that, with few exceptions, the food served is simple (see Regional

American, page 9). On all routes, avoid the snacks like potato chips, cookies, soft drinks, and candy, all of which are loaded with sugar and/or saturated fat.

Keep an eye on your food as well as on the scenery!

ON THE ROAD AGAIN

Finding an acceptable restaurant is often a challenge on a car trip, particularly in less-populated areas. However, you can always stop at a local market for an inexpensive supply of fruits, vegetables, and juices, yogurt, or even a sandwich. Lunch can be a picnic outdoors at a roadside stop.

GUIDELINES FOR AVOIDING WEIGHT GAIN WHEN TRAVELING

1 Set weight control as a goal. Decide before you leave on the trip that you won't return with excess baggage in the form of added body weight.
2 Order broiled foods, not fried. Choose fish, poultry, and vegetables without sauces or added fat. Choose fruit for dessert.
3 Avoid room service. A walk to find a meal discourages unnecessary eating and burns off some calories.
4 Keep breakfast simple. Cold or hot cereal and fruit will supply bulk and will help you avoid excess calories, saturated fat, and cholesterol.
5 Order nonalcoholic beverages like mineral water and fruit juices. Beer, wine, and liquor mean more calories.
6 Walk whenever you can in order to maintain or even lose weight. You'll see more of the sights you are visiting and you'll return home feeling healthy.

You can receive basic information on staying healthy when traveling from the International Health

Care Service, 440 East 69th Street, New York, New York 10021. For $4.50, they will send you a booklet called *The International Health Care Traveler's Guide.*

HEALTHFUL TRAVEL TALK

More and more people today are traveling far and wide. Since it is easier to get what you want if you make your requests in the language of the country you are visiting, I have prepared—with the help of Carol and Raphael Buitrago and Lore Zeller—a list of phrases and questions to use when ordering food in several foreign countries. If you are shy about trying to speak, you can simply show the appropriate phrase to your waiter.

FRENCH

I'm on a special low-fat, low-cholesterol diet.

Je suis un régime special sans matières grasses et sans cholesterol.

Do you have a soup that is not creamed?

Est-ce-que vous avez de la soupe sans crème?

Please serve my food plain, no sauce, gravy, or added fat or butter, please.

S'il vous plaît, je voudrai ce plat sans sauce, sans graisse, et sans beurre.

I cannot eat eggs.

Je ne peux pas manger des oeufs.

No fried foods, please.

Pas de fritures, s'il vous plaît.

May I have this food:.
broiled/grilled?
boiled?
steamed?
without butter or fat?

Pourriez-vous me préparer ce plat:
sur le grille (grillé)?
bouilli?
à la vapeur?
sans beurre ni graisse?

No butter, cheese, or cream sauces, please.

S'il vous plaît, pas de beurre ni de sauces à la crème.

Do you have:

Est-ce-que vous avez:

skim milk?

du lait écremé?

fresh fruit?

des fruits frais?

salad?

une salade?

steamed vegetables?

des vegetables à la vapeur

I want:

Je voudrais:

a fish dish.

du poisson.

a chicken dish.

du poulet.

May I have:

Avez-vous:

a fruit plate (with plain yogurt)?

un plat de fruit (avec du yaourt simple)?

pasta or noodles (without eggs) with tomato and herbs or vegetables?

des pâtes (sans oeufs) avec des tomates, des herbes, ou des verdures?

Can this dish be prepared without added salt?

Est-ce-que vous pouvez préparer ce plat sans sel?

SPANISH

I'm on a special low-fat, low-cholesterol diet.

Sigo una dieta especial, baja en grasas y colesterol.

Do you have a soup that is not creamed?

Hay una sopa que no tiene crema?

Please serve my food plain, no sauce, gravy, added fat or butter, please.

Por favor, quisiera la comida simple, sin salsas, grasas, o mantequilla.

I cannot eat eggs.

No puedo comer huevos.

No fried foods, please.

Nada de comida frita, por favor.

May I have this food:
broiled?
grilled?
boiled?
steamed?
without butter or fat?

Por favor, me podrían preparar este plato:
asado?
a la brasa?
hervido?
al vapor?
sin mantequilla o grasa?

No butter, cheese, or cream sauces, please.
Sin salsas, mantequilla, queso, o crema, por favor.

Do you have:
Hay:
skim milk?
leche descremada?
fresh fruit?
fruta fresca?
salad?
ensalada
steamed vegetables?
legumbres al vapor

I want:
Quisiera:
a fish dish.
un plato de pescado
a chicken dish.
un plato de pollo.

May I have:
Por favor, quisiera:
a fruit plate (with plain yogurt)?
un plato de frutas (con yoghurt)?
pasta or noodles (without eggs) with tomato and herbs or vegetables?
pasta (sin huevo) con salsa de tomato y hierbas o con verduras?

Can this dish be prepared without added salt?
Se puede preparar esto plato sin sal?

I'm on a special low-fat, low-cholesterol diet.

Io seguo una dieta speciale senza grassi e senza colesterolo.

Do you have a soup that is not creamed?

Avete una zuppa senza crema?

Please serve my food plain, no sauce, gravy, added fat, or butter, please.

Per favore prepara il mio cibo senza salsa, senza burro o grasso aggiunto.

I cannot eat eggs.

No posso mangiare uova.

No fried foods, please.

Per favore nessun cibo fritto.

May I have this food:
broiled/grilled?
boiled?
steamed?
without butter or fat?

Potrei aver questo:
ai ferri?
bolitto?
al vapore?
senza burro o grasso?

No butter, cheese, or cream sauces, please.

Per favore nessuna salsa con crema e niente burro.

Do you have:

Avete:

skim milk?

latte scremato?

fresh fruit?
frutta fresca?
salad?
insalata?
steamed vegetables?
legumi cotto al vapore?

I want:
Voglio:
a fish dish.
un piatto di pesce.
a chicken dish.
un piatto di pollo.
May I have:
Potrei avere:
a fruit plate (with plain yogurt)?
un piatto di frutta (con yogurt semplice)?
pasta or noodles (without eggs) with tomato and herbs or vegetables?
pasta (senza uovi) con pomodoro, spezie, o verdura?

Can this dish be prepared without added salt?
Si puo avere questo piatto senza sale?

GERMAN

I'm on a special low-fat, low-cholesterol diet.
Ich bin auf einer Diät ohne Fett, mit geringem Cholestrin Gehalt.

Do you have a soup that is not creamed?
Haben Sie eine Suppe ohne Sahne?

Please serve my food plain, no sauce, gravy, added fat, or butter, please.
Bitte richten Sie mein Essen an ohne Zutaten. Keine sauce, keine Fett, keine Butter, bitte.

I cannot eat eggs.

Ich darf keine Eier essen.

No fried foods, please.

Nichts Gebratenes, bitte.

May I have this food:
broiled/grilled?
boiled?
steamed?
without butter or fat?

Kann ich dies:
gegrillt haben?
gekocht haben?
gedünstet haben?
ohne Butter oder Fett haben?

No butter, cheese, or cream sauces, please.

Bitte keine Butter, keine Käse, Keine Fettsaucen.

Do you have:

Haben Sie:

skim milk?

Magermilch?

fresh fruit?

frisches Obst?

salad?

Salat?

steamed vegetables?

Gedünstet Gemüse?

I want:

Ich moechte:

a fish dish.

Fisch essen.

a chicken dish.

Huhn oder Geflügel.

May I have:

Kann ich:

a fruit plate (with plain yogurt)?

eine Fruchtplatte mit Yogurt (ohne Zutaten) haben?

pasta or noodles (without eggs) with tomato and herbs or vegetables?

Teigwaren oder Nudeln (ohne Ei) mit Tomaten, Kräutern, oder Gemüse haben?

Can this dish be prepared without added salt?

Kann dieses Gericht ohne extra Salz angerichtet werden?

So, I'll close with a *Bon appétit!*
Buen provecho!
Bon appetito!
Guten Appetit!